A New You
Healthy eating and weight management guide

By

Amanda Johnson

MSc, BSc (hons), PG Dip Diet

DEDICATION

Dedicated to all my amazing clients who over the years have
lost hundreds of kilograms between them, and who have
gone on to lead fitter, healthier, happier lives.

CONTENTS

1 Are you a healthy weight?   6

2 Food and nutrition   13

3 The practical stuff when it comes   28
   to food

4 Fad diets   39

5 Physical activity   47

6 Food and behaviour   54

7 Putting it all together   73

1: ARE YOU A HEALTHY WEIGHT?

Overweight and obesity are common across the world. In fact, in many developed countries now, more than half the population are above the healthy weight range.

Being obese is associated with a number of health problems (page 7), but by losing weight and attaining a healthy weight, it has been estimated that you can add up to 10 years to your lifespan.

Your health is important and by improving your diet and lifestyle you can add years to your life and life to your years, enjoying a better quality of life for longer.

Whether you want to maintain a healthy weight; lose weight because you are overweight or obese; or whether you simply want to trim down a little, you are what you eat, and good nutrition is very important to your short-term well-being and to your longer-term health. As the list on page 7 shows, there are a number of quite serious health problems that are linked to being obese.

Table 1: Major health risks associated with obesity

Adult-onset diabetes	Breathing problems
Heart disease	Varicose veins
Stroke	Hernias
High blood pressure	Dermatitis
High cholesterol	Sleep problems
Cancer	Reproductive problems
Back pain	
Arthritis	Pregnancy complications
Gout	Surgery complications
	Depression

How do I know if I am a healthy weight, overweight or obese?

BMI

Body mass index (BMI) is an index measurement that was first developed by a Belgium astronomer called Quetelet, who noticed that in adults of normal build, weight was proportional to height. It is calculated by dividing weight in kg by height in m^2.

For most people their body mass index will range between 20 and 40. The figure that applies to you can then be translated into the level of risk to your health.

What will you need?

(a) You will need an accurate set of scales to measure your weight. If you don't have a set of scales visit your local pharmacy, gym or health centre. Weigh yourself without shoes and wearing just light indoor clothing. You need to know your weight in kilograms.

(b) You will then need to work out your height in metres. If you are not sure just pop down to your local health centre or gym and ask to be measured.

(c) Now you can simply calculate your personal BMI figure, and find out which category you fall into.

BMI = Weight (kg) ÷ Height (m²)

BMI – what does it mean?

BMI under 18.5

If your BMI is less than 18.5 you are underweight and may benefit from gaining some weight. Talk to your GP or to a nutritionist or dietitian for more specific individual advice.

BMI 18.5 to 25

You are the ideal weight for your health. Don't forget to keep up good eating habits and take regular exercise.

BMI 25 to 29

You are overweight, but not clinically obese. At this level there is a slightly increased risk to health. If you are towards the upper end of this range you may wish to consider losing weight, as there is a risk you may tip over into the obese category.

BMI 30 to 39

You are classed as clinically obese. At this level you may find you have little energy and tire easily, becoming short of breath. This is because of the burden of the excess weight you are carrying around. You are at increased risk of ill health because of your weight. You should seriously consider losing weight and the information in this guide will help you achieve this.

BMI Over 40

You are classed as morbidly obese. Your weight means the risk to your health is extremely high. You would benefit enormously from losing weight. The information in this book will certainly help you, and will increase your understanding of the issues involved. You may also find it useful to seek specialised personal advice from a nutritionist or dietitian.

Body mass index is a useful measurement for all ages of people and for both sexes; it does however have some drawbacks. For those who are very muscular, body builders for example, a person may have a high body mass index without an increased risk to health. For most of us though, this is certainly a useful indication of health risk.

Waist circumference

Scientific evidence has suggested that simply measuring the size of your waist can be enough to tell you if your weight is a risk to your health. This is a much simpler measurement than body mass index.

To measure your waist use a cloth measuring tape and

relax (don't suck in your stomach); measure against your skin (not over clothes) and measure at about where your belly button is. You should do this while standing. Compare your waist measurement to the figures in the table below to see if you need to lose some weight.

Table 2: Health risk and waist circumference

	HEALTH RISK	
	INCREASED RISK	SUBSTANTIAL RISK
MEN	97cm to 102cm	102cm or more
WOMEN	80cm to 88cm	88cm or more

The solution

The key to long-term weight management really is adopting a healthy food intake and a healthy lifestyle. Essentially this means eating a balance of healthy foods – lots of fruits and vegetables, and not too many fatty or sugary foods – and taking regular physical activity. While weight-reducing, portion sizes should be a little smaller, then once you reach your target weight you simply upsize your portions a little.

Energy balance

Energy is another word for 'calories'; and balancing your energy is all about making sure that your **'energy in'** from food is balanced with your **'energy out'** from basic metabolism and keeping the body functioning (for example, breathing and heart beating), from the thermic effect of food (the amount of energy expended in digesting food) and from physical activity.

- **When energy consumed exceeds energy expended, you gain weight.**

- **When energy consumed is less than energy expended, you lose weight.**

You don't need to be in balance every single day – it is the general balance over time that will ensure you maintain your weight effectively.

This concept is illustrated in the diagram below.

Figure 1: Energy balance

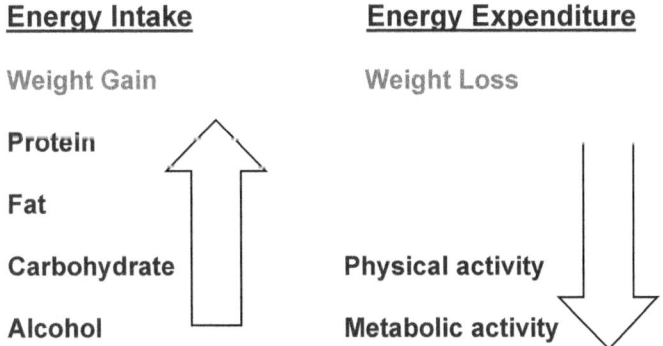

Energy Intake   **Energy Expenditure**

Weight Gain   Weight Loss

Protein

Fat

Carbohydrate   **Physical activity**

Alcohol   **Metabolic activity**

It's all about food, activity and behaviour

The key to success is to consider:

- **Food**
- **Activity**
- **Behaviour**

This is called the **FAB** approach to weight management, and by thinking about all three areas you are much more likely to succeed. Having the right food is very important, so is staying physically active. But it is also very important to give careful consideration to behaviours around food and the motivation for eating.

The following chapters outline some key information and strategies for each of these areas to help get you on the road to success.

2: FOOD AND NUTRITION

This chapter is essentially all about teaching you healthier new eating habits. So you will lose weight if you need to and more importantly will maintain a healthy weight in the longer term. Dietary regimens that encourage you to eat a pre-determined list of foods are unlikely to work in the long term, as you won't be able to stick to it forever. It is much better to use your current diet as a starting point and to modify this to make it healthier.

By taking this approach you will be able to adapt your new healthy diet to fit well with your family situation and lifestyle so is much more likely to work. It is suitable not just for those who are overweight, but for everyone, to optimise health status and to reduce risk of chronic disease later in life. If you are weight reducing you simply have smaller portions.

Calorie counting is to be discouraged; the best philosophy is to aim for a balanced and varied diet based on lots of fruits and vegetables, which is low in fat. Also, it is important to remember that are no good or bad foods; it is the overall balance of the diet that is important, so if you want to eat chips and chocolate you can, as long as it is only as an occasional treat and forms a small proportion of your diet.

Rate of weight loss

Most people who need to lose weight want to lose it as quickly as possible: that's why the fad diets and instant cures are so popular. However, if you want to maintain that loss, you need realistic goals and an eating pattern that you can stick to. Aim to shed 0.25–1 kg per week (0.5–2 lbs), which is equivalent to 13–52 kg per year (2–8 stone), until you reach your target weight. This is slower than many people would like, but remember that you are probably reducing weight much faster than you gained it in the first place.

Eating patterns

Some diets recommend a particular eating pattern as a way of increasing the metabolic rate and, therefore, helping weight loss. Some people propose eating lots of small meals; others advise three main meals in a day. But who is right? The scientific research into this area suggests that the meal patterns you adopt have very little effect on your metabolic rate. It is unlikely that they affect your weight either up or down. The best advice is to do what suits you, your family situation and your lifestyle. If you like to have lots of small snacks and light meals, that's just fine. If you prefer to have just three meals a day and nothing in-between, that's OK too. The most important consideration is the overall food intake throughout the day, so don't be drawn into a change just because it's the latest fad.

Basic nutrition

Most of who have watched our weight have a fairly good understanding of basic nutrition. However, there can sometimes be some confusion of the more complex terms. Most of us like to work with calories for example, as a measure of energy, but most food labels are in kilojoules, what's the difference you may ask? Well this is explained below. Also, you may find information on the different types of fatty acids useful, which ones are better, how many calories are in each? The following guide runs through in simple terms some basic nutrition facts that are useful for anyone following a weight reducing regimen or simply looking to have a healthy diet.

Energy

We get energy from food. Our bodies use it for activity, or store it. You will no doubt have noticed that different units are used for energy values. The most popular unit is the calorie, which is short for kilocalorie (kcal). The term used on food labels is kilojoule (kJ), although kcal may be given as well.

In order to convert kJ into kcal, use the following formula:

kcal = kJ divided by 4.2

In other words, a kcal has roughly a quarter of the value of a kJ.

As a guide, the average daily energy requirement for a woman is about 2000 kcal, and for a man about 2500 kcal. It is important to remember that these are just average figures and do not apply to everyone. A petite and inactive woman will have a much lower energy requirement than one who is tall and active. However, if you reduce your daily calorie intake to 500–1000 kcal below requirements, this should result in a weight loss of 0.5–1 kg (1–2 lbs) per week.

Carbohydrates

At least half of our energy intake should be provided by carbohydrate foods. Reducing the amount of fat in the diet and increasing the proportion of carbohydrate is likely to reduce energy intake, as carbohydrate provides about half as many calories as fat. There is no scientific evidence to support the low-carbohydrate, high-fat diets as a way of losing weight; studies have shown that weight loss following this type of diet is usually re-gained.

A low glycaemic index diet that is high in unrefined carbohydrates can have a positive impact on health, particularly for those at risk of excess weight, heart disease and Type 2 diabetes.

Starches

Starchy foods include potatoes, bread, breakfast cereals, rice and pasta. These should be the main sources of energy in our diets; they also provide B vitamins, and wholegrain varieties provide dietary fibre. It is important to avoid adding too much fat to carbohydrate foods (e.g., butter in potatoes, potato chips that are fried, butter on bread). Stay away from high-fat breads such as croissants, and have pita or a bread roll instead. Wholegrain varieties can help to fill you up.

Sugars

Sugar is a general term for a number of sweet-tasting substances including sucrose (table sugar), fructose (fruit sugar), lactose (milk sugar) and glucose. If you have a sweet tooth, there is no harm in including a little sugar in your diet — for example, a scraping of jam on your toast or the occasional dessert. If you do wish to have sugary treats, have them as part of a meal and brush your teeth afterwards. Sucking sweets or drinking high-sugar beverages constantly throughout the day can have an adverse effect on your teeth and can push up your energy intake.

Dietary fibre

A good intake of fibre is important for the proper functioning of the gut and can reduce risk of some chronic diseases; for example heart disease, cancer and diabetes. Dietary fibre is essentially the part of the plant that is resistant to digestion and absorption in the human body. Dietary fibre promotes laxation (going to the toilet), soluble fibre can help reduce blood cholesterol and fibre can also help modulate blood glucose levels. The suggested dietary intake is 28g per day in adult women and 38g per day in adult men. Children and adolescents need less.

Glycaemic index

Glycaemic Index (GI) is a way of ranking carbohydrate foods based on the rate at which they raise blood glucose levels. GI ranks foods from 0 to 100.

- Foods with a GI of over 70 are considered high GI
- Foods with a GI of 55-70 are considered medium GI
- Foods below 55 are considered low GI.

Foods with a high GI produce a rapid rise in blood glucose levels after eating, whereas low GI foods produce a much more gradual rise in the blood glucose.

A low GI diet may be helpful for people with diabetes and insulin resistance, since blood glucose levels are likely to be more stable than when high GI foods are consumed. Low GI foods may also help with weight control and blood lipid levels.

GI is not the only criteria that should be considered when selecting foods to include in a healthy diet. Choosing foods low in fat is also important. Also, you should remember that some low GI foods are not necessarily the best choice. Chocolate has a medium GI, owing to its fat content, and crisps have a lower GI than potatoes cooked without fat. Watermelon, bread, rice and potatoes are all high GI foods but can be eaten as part of a healthy diet. Starchy foods with a high GI include potatoes and some breakfast cereals. Foods with a low GI include pasta, oats and lentils.

As well as considering the type of food eaten, the GI of a food can be influenced by the cooking method, the amount of processing it has undergone, and the other foods eaten with it. For example, eating cheese with bread produces a lower GI than eating the bread on its own. Furthermore, the effects vary from individual to individual. Further information on the GI of different foods can be found at www.glycemicindex.com.

Putting it into practice

- Have at least one low GI food at each meal.
- Use a low GI bread and cereal, and include pasta and legumes in your diet.
- Keep foods 'whole', for example wholegrain rather than wholemeal or white bread, whole fruit rather than juice and raw, unpeeled fruit and vegetables where possible.

Table 3: Substituting low GI foods for high GI foods

High GI food	Lower GI food
Bread: whole wheat bread, white bread, French bread, white scones	Wholegrain bread (such as 100% stone-ground) or sourdough bread e.g. Burgen bread, Vogels, Molenberg, Tip Top Goodness 9 grains, Linseed and soy, fruit bread. Choose the heavier dense breads.
Highly processed breakfast cereals (such as Coco Pops, cornflakes, rice bubbles)	Alternative breakfast cereals such as All-Bran, traditional rolled oats, Guardian, Special K
Cakes, biscuits, crackers, doughnuts, pastries, white scones.	Fruit: whole fresh fruit, Burgen fruit bread, Arnott's Vita Wheat crisp bread.
Mashed potatoes, white long grain rice, Jasmine rice	Pasta, legumes (such as chickpeas, cannellini beans or lentils), noodles, Basmati rice, Uncle Ben's Express rice, baby new potatoes with skin, jacket potatoes with skin.

Protein

Protein is needed for the growth and repair of body tissues. Protein-containing foods include meat, fish, eggs, milk and cheese. Protein can also be found in non-animal foods such as cereals, pulses and nuts, which are particularly useful sources for those on a vegan diet.

Most of us eat plenty of protein, so beware of the fad diets that promote high intakes. Also, watch out for any fat that may accompany a high protein food, choose lean meat or cut off and discard all the fat and choose low fat dairy products. Protein foods can help to promote satiety, or a feeling of fullness so include moderate amounts in your diet. However, most people do not need to be eating protein shakes, whey supplements or protein sports bars – these foods simply add extra energy to your diet and make it hard to shift the excess weight. Professional athletes should consult a specialist sports dietitian for specific advice on protein intakes – for the rest of us our protein requirements will be met by having a healthy balanced diet.

Fat

We need a small amount of fat in our diets to provide fat-soluble vitamins and essential fatty acids, but many of us eat far more fat than we actually need. This is the number-one nutrient to target for reduction. Fat contains twice as many calories as carbohydrate and protein, and all types of fat, whether saturated or unsaturated, contain the same number of calories. Just by adding fat to food it is possible to double the calorie content.

Some people are concerned that cutting down on fat could leave them deficient in essential fatty acids. In fact, this is almost impossible, as such small amounts are actually required. So the focus should certainly be to cut down on fat for optimal health and weight loss. Not only is it important to reduce total fat intake, but you should also consider the types of fatty acids in your diet. An explanation of these, and their sources, is given below.

Saturated fatty acids

These can raise the level of cholesterol in the blood, increasing the risk of heart disease. Fats that are hard tend to contain a higher proportion of saturated fatty acids. The main sources include:

- Animal fats such as butter, hard table margarine, cheese, chicken skin and meat fat.
- Pies, pastries, potato crisps, cakes and biscuits.
- Palm oil and coconut oil.

Trans fatty acids

Trans fatty acids are produced during food processing, for example of hard table margarines. We consume smaller amounts of these fats than of saturated fatty acids. However, this type of fat can also raise cholesterol levels and so increase the risk of heart disease; they should be kept to a minimum in the diet. Sources of *trans* fatty acids include:

- Hard table margarines.
- Cakes, pastries and biscuits.
- Beef, lamb, milk and dairy fat.

Mono-unsaturated fatty acids

Mono-unsaturated fatty acids are a healthier form of fat, and can be used to replace the saturated fatty acids. The main sources are olive oil and rapeseed (canola) oil. Look out for the fat spreads based on these oils. Other sources are nuts, lean meat, chicken, eggs and fish.

Polyunsaturated fatty acids

These are also a healthier form of fat. There are two types. Omega-6 helps to reduce blood cholesterol levels. The main sources are sunflower and soybean oil, soft margarines, nuts and seeds. Omega-3 helps to reduce the tendency of the blood to clot, and may help to protect against heart disease. The main sources of the omega-3 fatty acids are oily fish such as herring, mackerel, salmon and sardines.

Cutting back

Your intake of saturated and *trans* fatty acids should be kept to a minimum. Always trim the fat from meat and remove the skin from chicken, choose lower fat dairy products, and either avoid or only eat a very limited amount of pies, cakes, biscuits, and hard spreads such as butter, lard and hard margarine.

Don't forget that all types of fat contain the same number of calories. However, by changing from saturated and *trans* fatty acids to the mono- and polyunsaturated fatty acids, you will make your diet much healthier, and reduce the risk of raised cholesterol and heart disease. All the same, do remember that you should not be increasing your intake of fat or pouring excessive amounts of oil over your foods. Try some of these suggestions:

- Bake your own cakes using the healthier types of fat, or eliminate the fat.
- Choose low-fat spreads and oils based on mono- or polyunsaturated fatty acids.
- Use spray oils based on mono- and polyunsaturated fats, to minimise the amount of fat.
- Include at least two portions a week of oily fish.

Alcohol

Alcohol can be a significant source of calories. Too much alcohol can also be a risk to our health. New recommendations suggest that if you do drink, women should drink no more than one standard drink a day, and men no more than two standard drinks a day.

We should, of course, have some drink-free days. Women who may become pregnant or who are pregnant or breastfeeding are advised to avoid alcohol completely. One standard drink is equal to 10g of alcohol, which is the amount in 285mls of full strength beer, 100mls of wine or 30mls of spirits.

Vitamins and minerals

Vitamins and minerals are important for good health. A balanced diet should provide all the vitamins and minerals we need. The role they play, and common food sources, are listed here.

Table 4: Function and sources of vitamins and minerals

Vitamin/mineral	Function	Sources
Vitamin A	Aids growth and development, immune function, night vision.	Liver, kidney, whole milk, margarine. Carotenoids found in carrots, red and orange fruit and dark green vegetables can be converted into vitamin A in the body.
Vitamin D	Important for healthy bones.	Oily fish, fortified foods such as margarine and breakfast cereals. Can also be produced by the body on exposure to sunlight.
Vitamin E	Acts as an antioxidant and is involved in immune function.	Vegetable oils, wholegrain cereals, dark green vegetables and nuts.
Vitamin K	Needed for clotting of the blood and bone health.	Green leafy vegetables, some fruit, vegetable oils and cereals.

Vitamin B1 (thiamin)	Involved in metabolism.	Cereals and potatoes. Some in meat, poultry and nuts.
Vitamin B2 (riboflavin)	Involved in metabolism.	Milk and milk products, fortified cereals. Some in meat and meat products.
Vitamin B3 (niacin)	Involved in metabolism.	Meat and meat products, bread, fortified cereals, potatoes, milk and milk products.
Vitamin B6	Involved in metabolism.	Potatoes and breakfast cereals.
Vitamin B12	Metabolism of folate, involved in the nerves.	Only found naturally in foods of animal origin, e.g., meat, meat products and milk. Often added to breakfast cereals.
Folate (folic acid)	Involved in metabolism. Helps development of the neural tube in unborn babies.	Wholegrain cereals, liver, leafy green vegetables.
Vitamin C	Needed for wound healing, healthy skin, a healthy immune system. Helps the absorption of iron from vegetable sources.	Citrus fruit, berry fruit, salad vegetables, peppers, potatoes.
Iron	Needed for healthy red blood cells, growth and development in young children.	Red meat, fish, fortified cereals, pulses and nuts. Plant sources are poorly absorbed.

Calcium	Needed for healthy strong bones and teeth.	Milk and dairy products, canned fish eaten with bones, fortified breads and cereals.

Antioxidants

Antioxidants have had a lot of coverage in the popular press, but what exactly do they do, and where can you find them? Well, they are substances that help to prevent oxidation reactions in the body. Oxidation reactions are thought to be linked to ageing and the development of chronic diseases such as cancer and heart disease. Some vitamins and minerals have antioxidant effects — for example, vitamin C, vitamin E and carotenoids (which are converted to vitamin A in the body), selenium, manganese, zinc and copper.

New research shows that there is a whole range of other chemicals in plants that may also have antioxidant activity in the body, for example, flavonoids found in red wine, and some fruit and vegetables, and lycopene found in tomatoes.

It is important to remember that there are hundreds of chemicals in a piece of fruit or in a vegetable, in a particular amount and combination. Although we know that eating fruit and vegetables is beneficial, and that part of the effect may be the presence of antioxidants, we do not yet know enough to recommend taking antioxidant supplements. These may in fact have adverse effects, particularly at high doses. Until there is much more large-scale research on humans, the current advice is to eat lot of fruit and vegetables and to stay away from high-dose antioxidant supplements.

Supplements

The use of nutrient supplements is common; however, the best nutritional strategy for most people to promote optimal health and reduce the risk of chronic disease is to consume a healthy balanced diet based on a wide variety of foods. For some people though, extra nutrients in the form of supplements can help meet nutritional needs - such as when there is a diagnosed deficiency of a nutrient or when nutrient needs are increased.

Groups within the population most vulnerable to nutrient inadequacy include some older adults, pregnant women, people who are food insecure (or who are unable to buy enough food), people who are alcohol dependant, strict vegetarians and vegans, and those with increased needs due to a health condition.

- Pregnant women:

Folic acid reduces the risk of having a baby with a neural tube defect. It is recommended that a folic acid supplement of 800µg (0.8mg) per day is taken by women for 4 weeks before conception and 12 weeks afterwards. Pregnant and breastfeeding women also have high iodine requirements and should take a daily 150µg iodine supplement to help meet their iodine requirements.

- Vegans

Vegans (who eliminate all animal products from the diet) are advised to take a vitamin B12 supplement. They may also need iron and calcium supplements.

- Milk avoiders

For those who consume little or no milk products a calcium supplement may be necessary.

- Iron deficiency

For diagnosed iron-deficiency anaemia, iron supplementation may be warranted.

- Low sun exposure

For people with low sunlight exposure, and for housebound people, particularly the elderly, a vitamin D supplement may be necessary.

High doses

Some vitamins have been associated with adverse effects at high doses. For example, excess folic acid may exacerbate a deficiency of vitamin B12.

High dose antioxidant nutrients consistently show either no benefit or an adverse effect. An example of adverse effect is an increase in lung cancer, which has been found in people taking beta-carotene supplements.

Fat soluble vitamins are not readily excreted from the body. Particular care should be taken if multiple supplement products are being consumed that intakes do not become excessive. Vitamin A (in the form of retinol), for example, is teratogenic (can cause birth defects) and pregnant women are advised to avoid vitamin A supplements.

Taking too much of one nutrient can also affect the body's use of other nutrients. For example, high doses of iron supplements can inhibit copper absorption, and absorption of iron can be inhibited by calcium. Also, the nutrients supplied by supplements may be less bioavalable than those supplied by foods.

The latest advice on supplements

Having a nutrition supplement does not compensate for a poor diet as the supplement may top up only some of the nutrients inadequately supplied by food. Also, there are many beneficial substances in foods that would be difficult to package into a pill; for example fibre and various phytochemicals. We have yet to identify all the types and amounts of biologically active components in foods, so it would not be possible to get all the benefits of food into a 'pill'! Nutrient imbalances and toxicity are much less likely if we consume our nutrients as foods. For those with a genuine need for an extra intake of a particular nutrient, supplements should be taken as prescribed or recommended by a doctor or nutritionist (or health professional). For those who wish to take a supplement as an insurance policy to ensure they are getting everything they need, then it is best to choose a general multi vitamin/mineral supplement that provides a wide range of nutrients at levels that are around the 'recommended daily intake'. Mega-dosing or taking multiple supplements is not recommended.

3 THE PRACTICAL STUFF WHEN IT COMES TO FOOD

The basics

The key recommendations from experts are to eat well by including a variety of foods in the diet every day, based on the four main food groups.

- Have lots of fruit and vegetables, which provide fibre and important vitamins and minerals. Aim for **at least** five portions a day (a portion is approximately a handful).
- Include plenty of bread, cereals (especially wholegrains) which provide energy.
- Consume moderate amounts of lean meat, fish, eggs, pulses and/or nuts, to provide iron.
- Eat moderate amounts of lower-fat milk and dairy foods, which provide calcium.

Foods and drinks should be prepared with minimal fat (especially saturated fat), salt and sugar. We should have plenty of fluids every day – especially water; and alcohol intakes should be limited.

Maintaining a healthy body weight can be achieved by choosing the right amounts of healthy foods and maintaining physical activity.

Getting the right balance

Shopping

Buying the right foods is a basic first step in establishing a new pattern of eating. Then by preparing and cooking these foods so that the fat content is minimised and the balance is right, you can be confident that you are on the road to success.

However, it's all too easy to buy the wrong things in the supermarket, with the aisles full of tempting products and packets. At this time, more than any other, it's important to be disciplined and to buy the right foods. There are a few basic tips that can help you with your shopping:

- Never shop when you are hungry, this will just lead you to buy all the wrong foods.

- Always make a shopping list, and try to stick to it.

- If you have a real weakness for a particular food (such as chocolate, potato chips or cheese) to the extent that you know that you will just binge on it, then don't buy it. If it isn't in the house you can't eat it during a weak moment. Select other treats instead.

- Sometimes it's easy to just skip the isle with the chocolates, confectionary and biscuits, if this helps you to stay away from temptation then do it!

- If possible, go shopping on your own, children can be distracting and can tempt you into buying things you had not planned to purchase.

- Look carefully at the labels when you are buying foods to compare brands; go for the lowest fat options.

- Go to the Deli counter and buy as much as you need, rather than buying larger packs of pre-packaged foods.

What's on a label?

It helps to understand nutrition labelling. The food label usually lists the nutrients, often given per 100g and per serve, and there may also be nutrition claims. In most countries there are stringent regulations governing the claims that can be made on products.

Most commonly listed in the nutrient information are energy, protein, fat and carbohydrate. Saturated fatty acids, sugars, fibre and sodium (salt) may also be listed.

Sometimes there are details on cholesterol, starch, mono-unsaturated fatty acids and polyunsaturated fatty acids, vitamins and minerals, particularly if there are claims in relation to these.

Here are some tips on what to look for on a food label.

- Use the per 100g information to compare between products. Take note of the recommended serving size – if you have more than this you will be consuming more nutrients per serve

- Energy is usually given in kJ on food labels. To convert to kilocalories, divide this number by 4.2. On average, women need about 2000 calories (8400 kJ) per day and men need about 2500 calories (10500 kJ) per day. If you are on a weight reducing diet you will be aiming to consume less than this amount.

- For snack foods, aim for 100 to 150 kcal (420 to 630 kJ) per snack.

- Look out for yoghurts that contain less than 5g fat and less than 10g sugar per 150g pot.

- When choosing breakfast cereals go for lower GI options and look for varieties that provide more than 5g dietary fibre, less than 5g fat and less than 15g sugar per 100g. If some of the sugar comes from fruit – aim for less than 25g per 100g.

- It is recommended that about 15% of our energy comes from protein. This is about 75g for a woman and 95g for a man, per day, on average.

- Fat: In general, aim for foods with less than 10g total fat and 2g saturated fatty acids per 100g. Women should be aiming for less than 70g per day total fat and men less than 95g per day total fat. If you are following a weight reducing diet, your fat intake should be lower than this.

- When choosing a table spread – go for lower fat spreads and choose those that are high in monounsaturates or polyunsaturates, and low in saturates and *trans* fatty acids. Look for options that are less than 70g of total fat, less than 20g saturated fat, and less than 400mg sodium per 100g.

- Carbohydrate: Focus on wholegrains and low glycaemic index foods. The 'sugars' value should be minimal; in general look for products with less than 10-15g of sugar per 100g.

- Sodium: To convert sodium values on the food label to salt, multiply the sodium value by 2.5. Men should be having less than 7g salt per day and women less that 5g salt per day. Most of our salt intake is from processed foods – so as well as avoiding adding salt to foods, check the food labels. When choosing individual foods – aim for less than 0.3g (300mg) of sodium per serving.

- 'Best before' dates refer to the quality of a food. 'Use by' dates relate to the safely of a food – do not eat foods after the use by date.

Food preparation and cooking tips

Here are some suggestions for eating healthily when preparing and cooking food.

- Don't eat while preparing food.

- Don't be afraid to throw away food after the meal; or you can freeze or refrigerate leftovers. Eating leftovers to save waste won't save your waist.

- If you live alone, prepare meals for 4–6 and freeze into individual portions. This is a great way to have healthy 'ready-meals' when you rush in late from work.

- Always trim all the visible fat from meat.

- Remove and discard the skin from chicken and turkey either before cooking, or before serving.

- Buy lean bacon rather than streaky, and premium minced meat, rather then economy; it may be more expensive but it's best to spend the same amount of money and buy less. You save, as there is less waste.

- Try home-made burgers made with lean minced meat as an alternative to shop-bought or take-away varieties.

- Extend small amounts of lean meat with pulses (peas, beans, lentils) and lots of vegetables.

- Use lower fat yoghurt, milk and cheese.

- Grate cheese rather than slicing — it goes further and you need less.

- Use low fat yoghurt instead of cream.

- Make your own low-fat salad dressings lemon juice or vinegar along with herbs and spices.

- Dry-fry if possible to avoid adding extra fat to food, or just use a light spray of unsaturated oil.

- Grill foods on a rack so excess fat drains away.

- Skim fat off the top of casseroles and stews.

- Make your own low-fat oven chips or roast potatoes – just spray lightly with olive oil.

- Use skim milk rather than butter when mashing vegetables.

- Choose lower fat sauces and salad dressings, and avoid using too much.

- Have moist fillings in sandwiches to avoid the need for any fat spreads.

- Have dry toast with baked beans; no need for fat spreads here either.

- Have a thin scraping of jam on toast instead of butter.

- Use herbs and spices instead of salt.

- When baking:
  - Use small amounts of low fat spread (or use yoghurt instead, ¼ cup of yoghurt replaces 60g butter).
  - Use filo pastry brushed with milk instead of butter.
  - Reduce sugar and replace with dried or pureed fruit.
  - Replace coconut cream with lite evaporated milk.
  - Use wholegrain flour instead of white.

- Try serving on smaller plates and bowls to avoid the temptation of serving excessive portions.

Portion sizes

One area that causes a lot of confusion is the size of a portion. As food outlets offer increasingly generous servings in order to give good value for money, you can end up with much more than you want or need

We are becoming used to these over-sized helpings from a very young age. You and your family may need to re-assess what constitutes an appropriate serving. As a starting point it may be useful to purchase a set of scales and weigh out standard portions of food, just so you get an idea visually what a portion looks like. The table on the next pages shows portion sizes for different foods, classified into the different food groups.

Note: 1 cup is equivalent to 250 ml, or half a pint.

Table 5: Portion sizes

Food	Portion size
Fruit and vegetables	**Have at least 5 per day from a variety of sources**
Potato, kumara and root vegetables	1 medium (135 g)
Cooked vegetables, e.g., corn, peas, green beans	Half a cup (50–80 g)
Salad	Half a cup (60 g)
Tomato	1 medium (80 g)
Fruit, e.g., apple, pear, banana, orange	1 medium (130 g)
Stone fruit, e.g., apricot, plum	2 medium (100 g)
Fruit salad/stewed (fresh or tinned)	Half a cup (120 g)
Stewed fruit	Half a cup (135 g)
Fruit juice	1 cup

Breads and cereals	Choose wholegrain varieties. Aim for 6-11 servings depending on your target energy intake.
1 small bread roll	50 g
1 medium slice of bread	30 g
1 small pita bread	50 g
Cornflakes	1 cup (30 g)
Muesli	Half a cup (55 g)
Weetbix or Weetabix	Two biscuits (35 g)
Cooked cereal, e.g., porridge	Half a cup (130 g)
Cooked pasta	1 cup (150 g)
Cooked rice	1 cup (150 g)
Milk and milk products	Have at least 2 servings a day and choose the lower fat varieties.
Milk	1 cup
Yoghurt	1 pot (150 g)
Cheese	Matchbox-sized piece (40 g)

Meat, fish and alternatives	Have 1-2 servings a day and trim off all visible fat.
Cooked meat e.g., ham or chicken	2 slices (100 g)
Eggs	1 medium (50 g)
Beans	¾ cup
Steak	1 medium (120 g)
Chicken drumsticks	2 (110 g)
Fillet of fish	1 (150g)
Nuts	2 Tbsp or ½ cup
Foods containing fats	Keep these to a minimum
Foods containing sugar	Don't eat these too frequently and limit your intake

Convenience foods and fast foods

Most of us couldn't manage without frozen, canned or packaged food. Sometimes these are criticised for being less healthy than fresh food, but there is actually nothing wrong with this option. However, fast foods can be high in fat, salt and sugar, so be careful where you go and what choices you make. Chips, pies and fried foods are all high in fat and salt; fizzy drinks and sweet treat foods are high in sugar. Instead choose sandwiches, pizzas with vegetable toppings (but go easy on the cheese), grilled fish or chicken sandwiches, filled jacket potatoes and salads.

Drink water and include fresh fruit with your meal.

Try making your own fast foods at home. It only takes about ten minutes to put together a stir-fry or some delicious low-fat burgers with oven chips. This is probably about how long you would spend waiting for your meal in a fast-food outlet or waiting for a take-away to be delivered.

Eating out

When you're in a restaurant, sometimes the best-laid plans can be challenged. Here are a few tips:

- Select restaurants and outlets that have healthy options.

- Try the sandwich shops that allow you to select your own ingredients.

- Stay away from calorie-laden nibbles such as nachos, prawn crackers and garlic bread.

- If you really have to take the kids to a burger bar, select a plain burger and ask for it to be prepared specially, with no mayonnaise. Some burger/fast food outlets have options that are lower in fat and energy and/or salads so make healthier choices where possible. Have water, a diet drink, a tea or a coffee to go with it.

- At buffet-type restaurants, go for the healthy options and visit the buffet bar only once.

- Don't be afraid to ask for information on what's in the different dishes and how they are served. Most restaurants will be happy to modify your meal for you to suit your needs.

- Order baked potato rather than fries, and extra vegetables or salad to fill you up.

- Choose plain rice or noodles rather than fried.

- If you are served a giant portion, don't be tempted to eat it all. Ask for the remainder to be packed up for you to take home.

- Avoid the temptation to 'super-size' your meal, it may seem like good value but you don't really want or need the extra food, as it will just pile on the weight.

Drinks

It's important to drink plenty of fluids, especially in hot weather and during heavy exercise, to replace that lost in sweat. The average adult needs at least 6–8 cups of fluid a day (1.5 litres or 2½ pints).

Water is one of the best options. Try the sparkling mineral waters for a change; add flavours such as lemon juice and mint leaves, or fruit such as oranges and lemons. Top up with ice and serve well chilled in an elegant glass.

Another option for a healthy drink is trim milk (green or yellow topped). Add fruit and low-fat ice cream for a delicious fruit smoothie. If you decide to have soft drinks, go for the low sugar or 'diet' versions.

4 FAD DIETS

Dieting is certainly big business. If you're struggling with your weight there is no end of options open to you, from the credible through to the wacky! At your local library or bookshop you'll find shelves full of titles offering to give you back eternal youth, to guarantee that you will lose weight if you follow their magic formula, to cleanse your body of toxins — the list goes on. Miracle diet books are certainly very believable. Often they use complex medical jargon, which could dupe even the most astute reader. There are also special foods, herbal preparations and even plasters that are claimed to help you lose weight.

Here are some of the signs to look out for that should make you very wary about wasting your money.

- Promises to solve your weight problem without having to change your lifestyle in any real way.

- Offers unlicensed and untested products such as herbal concoctions or hormones.

- Promises rapid weight loss of more than 1kg of body fat a week.

- Suggests special fat-burning effects of foods or supplements.

- Uses complex medical terminology and jargon to try and sound 'scientifically proven'.

- Promotes avoiding or severely limiting an entire food group, such as dairy products or a staple food such as wheat. It may also suggest substituting these foods with expensive doses of vitamin and mineral supplements.

- Promotes eating mainly one type of food (eg, cabbage soup, lemons, baby food, liquid foods) or avoiding all cooked foods (the raw food diet).

- Recommends eating foods only in particular combinations based on your genetic type or blood group.

- Suggests being overweight is related to a food allergy or a yeast infection.

- Recommends 'detoxing' or avoiding foods in certain combinations such as fruit with meals.

- Offers no supporting evidence apart from anecdotes from followers or even celebrities with a personal success story to tell.

Popular diets

Let's have a look at some of the diets on offer, and see which ones are likely to work, and which are just plain silly.

Detox Diets

Detox is certainly a popular buzzword in the dieting world! The idea behind it is that we need to periodically clear the "toxic waste" from our body in order to stay healthy. In particular, we might be tempted to detox after over-indulging a little, for example at Christmas. Some of the claims made in relation to detox diets include: rapid weight loss; improved digestion; improved hair, nails and skin; improved energy levels; boosted immune system; banishment of cellulite. Detox diets can last from around one day to around one month and may involve:

- Fasting for short periods of time.
- Consuming only fruits and vegetables.
- Cutting out wheat and dairy foods.
- Consuming a limited range of foods.
- Avoiding caffeine and alcohol.

Our body constantly filters out, breaks down and excretes toxins and waste products. These could include alcohol, medications, products of metabolism and digestion, dead cells, chemicals from pollution and bacteria. This is achieved by our in-built 'detoxifiers' the liver, the kidneys, skin, intestines and lungs. If we generally follow a healthy diet and lifestyle, they work in harmony to do the job rather well and we don't need special help.

Food combining

Dr William Hay developed the food-combining diet in the early 1900s. More recently it has re-emerged and a number of books advocating this approach have achieved great popularity. The theory is that you shouldn't eat carbohydrate foods (starches such as bread or rice, and sugars such as table sugar) at the same time as protein foods. Five rules are set out:

- Do not eat starches and sugars at the same time as proteins and acid fruits.
- Vegetables, salads and fruits should form the major part of the diet.
- Eat protein, starch and fat in small quantities.
- Eat only wholegrain and unprocessed starches. Avoid all refined and processed foods.
- Allow at least four hours between meals of different types.

Proponents of this diet claim that the digestive system works more effectively and that you will achieve weight loss and an improved health and well-being. This approach certainly won't do you any harm. You may even lose some weight as you grapple with the complex meal arrangements, and try to make them appetizing. Also, it's based on fruit, vegetables and whole grains, which we all know are good for us. The down side is as follows:

- There is absolutely no scientific evidence to support the concept. All the books are supported only by testimonials and anecdotes. Our bodies are, in fact, perfectly capable of digesting any combination of foods we may wish to consume.

- It's difficult to follow, and meals are unlikely to be appetising or interesting.
- In the longer term it's impossible to stick to.
- Any weight loss is due to a lower energy intake. In fact, you can achieve this with a sensible balanced diet.

The expert verdict on this one: don't waste your time, effort or money.

HcG Diet

This diet involves a very low calorie intake combined with hCG (human chorionic gonadotropin), a hormone found in the placenta during pregnancy. It is only licensed as a fertility drug, but is now being sold via the internet in a diluted 'homeopathic' form by the diet industry. The hCG diet is being promoted as a way of controlling the body's metabolism of fat, burning off long-term "abnormal" fat stores that (the promoters claim) are locked away and forgotten by the body. By having hCG (they claim) the body will burn this "abnormal" fat at a rate of 1-2lbs a day with no exercise.

The promise is that this hormone will trick your body into losing weight by reducing symptoms of hunger while you eat a very low-calorie diet (500 calories per day). This diet plan even claims to re-set your metabolism! Even more bizarre is the fact that for the first two days on this diet, people are encouraged to eat as much as they can, as often as they can, to promote fat storage in advance of the severe calorie restriction that follows.

In the USA, Canada, Europe, Australia and New Zealand, hCG is a prescription only medicine and has not been given approval to be used for any other purpose than fertility treatment, although products containing less than 10 parts per million may be imported into the country with no restriction, for example homeopathic drops.

This diet has been around for a long time. It was first promoted in the 1950s by Dr Simeons. Studies carried out since this time, have generally found that hCG is not an effective way to lose weight and have not recommended this as a weight loss approach.

In 1962, for example, an article in the *Journal of the American Medical Association* stated "continued adherence to such a drastic regimen is potentially more hazardous to a patient's health than continued obesity".

And in 1976 a double blind study published in *the American Journal of Clinical Nutrition,* which attempted to find out whether injecting hCG was an effective adjunct to a rigidly imposed dietary regimen for weight reduction, found no effect of hCG. The authors cast serious doubt on hCG as an effective weight loss tool.

In 2009 The American Society of Bariatric Physicians stated in a position statement that, "*Numerous clinical trials have shown HCG to be ineffectual in producing weight loss.*"They conclude that, "*The diet used in the Simeons method provides a lower protein intake than is advisable in view of current knowledge and practice. There are few medical literature reports favourable to the Simeons method; the overwhelming majority of medical reports are critical of it. Physicians employing either the hCG or the diet recommended by Simeons may expose themselves to criticism from other physicians, from insurers, or from government bodies.*"

So, steer well clear of this one.

Fasting and crash diets

Fasting, or severely restricting what you eat, limits intake of energy and important nutrients needed for health and well-being. Rapid weight loss can occur, but this weight loss is largely water and glycogen (the body's carbohydrate stores), rather than fat. You may feel fatigued and dizzy and it's likely you'll have less energy. Further, if you are fasting your body won't have the proper fuels available to carry out sustained exercise and activity – an important aspect of general well-being and healthy weight management. At the end of the programme, if you return to your old eating habits, any weight lost is likely to go back on!

Any regimen that involves consuming fewer than 800 kcal a day, can harmful as there would be a significant loss of lean body tissue. Such a restrictive regimen should only ever be followed following approval from a doctor and under close medical supervision.

Blood-group diets

This is truly one of the more weird approaches. The theory is that you should follow a particular diet depending on what blood group you are:

- **Type O**: eat meat and steer clear of wheat and most other grains.
- **Type A**: have a vegetarian diet.
- **Type B**: have a varied diet that includes meat. This is supposed to be the only blood type that does well with dairy products.
- **Type AB**: these are said to 'have most of the benefits and intolerances of types A and B'.

This theory is seriously flawed and there is no scientific evidence to back it up. There is a very high risk of ending up with a diet that is poorly balanced, or even deficient in some important nutrients. What's more, it would be pretty boring trying to follow some of the restrictive regimens.

Liver-cleansing diet

The theory behind the liver-cleansing diet is that excess weight and a sluggish metabolism are a result of an unhealthy liver. The eight-week 'liver-cleansing' plan involves following a gentle regimen for two weeks, followed by four weeks of a more serious cleansing plan, then a return to a less demanding plan for another two weeks. Recommended foods include raw fruit and vegetables, legumes, seeds, nuts, fish, free-range chicken and eggs.

Red meat is kept to a minimum and the advice is to avoid dairy products.

The truth of the matter is that this short-term diet will do little to actually cleanse the liver and there is no evidence that a poorly functioning liver leads to weight gain. Also, if you avoid dairy products, your calcium levels could be reduced, and there is also no evidence that meat has any adverse effect on the liver. However, the diet is based on healthy foods; fruits, vegetables and legumes are good for anyone, including those who are aiming to lose weight.

Zen macrobiotics

The philosophy of this diet is based on the principles of yin and yang (positive and negative) for optimum spiritual, mental and physical wellbeing. It involves a progression through ten levels, from a diet that is fairly well balanced to one consisting only of cereals. At this extreme the diet could actually be quite dangerous, as it's severely deficient in some nutrients.

One food diets - cabbage soup or grapefruit ...

We've all come across the one-food-only diet, where we are told that eating copious amount of a particular food will magically help us lose those extra kilos. While living solely on these foods will certainly help reduce your intake of calories, there is nothing magical about this. What's more, you won't be able to stick to them for very long and they won't be very enjoyable.

The solution

There is an easy solution to weight loss. It certainly doesn't involve following all sorts of funny combinations and permutations of food intake, although these types of regimens will be so difficult to follow they will probably lead to weight loss as you will be eating less. It's got nothing to do with any magical physiological effects, or any amazing metabolic boosting effects, it's just that reduction in energy intake. The simple solution is to reduce calorie intake and increase exercise. The challenge exists in putting this into practice; that's where the information in this guide on food will help you to get on the right track.

5 PHYSICAL ACTIVITY

Our ancestors had much more activity in their lives than we have today. Our grandmothers would have a multitude of daily chores such as washing the clothes by hand, milking the cows and churning the butter. Our grandfathers often cycled or walked to work and had professions that required physical activity, and this meant their level of energy expenditure was significant.

In today's modern society, we have changed the way we live with inventions such as cars, computers and dishwashers, along with a whole range of other labour saving devices. Also, many more people work in sedentary jobs, with the advent of computer technology. We even have remote controls for just about everything in the house these days so we don't even have to get out of our comfy armchairs to turn over the TV or change the CD. All these factors have all contributed to a lifestyle where we have to continually be creative in how we will burn energy.

Our bodies are designed to be active and the inactivity of today's culture can be viewed as an abnormal state that we need to reverse to avoid ill health and to achieve optimal functioning.

Activity levels

Your extra weight is made up of fat stores. The processes involved in gaining extra fat are extremely complex. However, one thing is certain: excess weight can only be gained when energy intake (what we eat) remains higher than energy expenditure (our activity), over an extended period of time. This is influenced by our biology, by our behaviour and by our environment. The key is to look not only at what we are eating but also at how active we are: and to lose weight, we need to expend more energy than we take in.

The risks of inactivity

Physical inactivity has been described as the fourth major risk factor for heart disease after smoking, high blood fats and high blood pressure. It can also put you at greater risk of other illnesses and being inactive can mean that you are twice as likely to die younger. So there's plenty of incentive to start moving.

Getting Started

Often, people worry about getting started with exercise, believing it will involve a major commitment in terms of time and energy. People are often relieved to find that just increasing activities such as walking and gardening could benefit them immensely. For these kinds of activities you wouldn't even need to change into any exercise gear, spend any money or involve anyone else.

The benefits of exercise

Not only does exercising and keeping fit reduce your health risks; it also brings a wide range of other benefits, for example:

- Helps in weight control.
- Reduces risk of high blood pressure.
- Aids management of Type 2 diabetes.
- Improves functional capacity.
- Favourably modifies blood fats.
- Reduces depression and anxiety.
- Improves self-esteem and well-being.
- Raises energy levels.
- Improves sleep.
- Helps to manage stress.
- Aids mental relaxation.
- Gives you a break from other areas of your life.
- Makes you feel great.

Types of movement

- Include more weight bearing movement as part of our daily lives e.g. walk up some or all of the stairs instead of taking a lift; make several trips a day up a sloped drive or a nearby road.

- Spend less time in sedentary pursuits such as watching TV and gradually make activity part of your daily lifestyle eg through gardening, walking the dog, walking to the shops or washing the car.

- Build up to bouts of gentle exercise sustained for 60 minutes or more at a time.

- Even though lower intensity activities burn less energy than more vigorous types of activity, it is likely to occur more frequently, be more sustainable and amount to a significant amount of energy expenditure over a period of weeks, months and years, and that's what we are aiming for. The ultimate aim is to both increase daily activity and to incorporate an extended period of physical activity into each day.

Taking action

It's time to have a look at the level of activity that's right for you. If you have a pre-existing medical condition or are concerned about your health, you are advised to consult your doctor before embarking on any exercise programme, particularly if you:

- Have not exercised seriously for over a year.
- Are obese.
- Have high blood pressure.
- Take any prescribed medication.
- Are a smoker.
- Are over 40 years of age.

Activity is very important in the life-long maintenance of your weight. It also keeps us fit, healthy and able to enjoy life to the full with our friends and family.

If you feel unwell or sustain injury as you start exercising, stop and seek medical advice.

Getting started

There are a few basic considerations before you really get going on your new lifestyle plan.

Do less than you think you can initially and don't be too over ambitious; setting goals that are not achievable will just set you up for failure.

- Build up slowly and gradually and start at a level that suits you, even if this is just a short walk or jogging session. Your aim though should be to initially build up to the equivalent of walking for at least 30 minutes (or even two fifteen minute sessions) on at least five days of the week.

- Once you have achieved a basic level of fitness, gradually extend some of your sessions to 45 to 60 minutes.

- Put more activity into your daily routine; walking up stairs, washing the car by hand, going shopping on foot, walking the dog, doing the gardening.

- Reduce the amount of time you spend in inactive leisure pursuits such as watching TV and replace these sedentary activities with more active pursuits.

- Begin by doing slightly more activity than you usually do, and building steadily. For example if you work on the eighth floor start by getting the lift to the seventh floor and walking up the last flight of stairs then add on one more floor as soon as you feel up to it until you are walking up all the stairs to your office at the beginning of each day. As you build confidence you will be able to increase the amount you do.

- There will be days where you will have aching muscles, or will feel tired, if this is the case have a rest and then continue with the exercise the next day. If you find you need a break from the more strenuous exercise, do some stretches, do a gentle walk or try some yoga. Once you feel ready to get back into your more active routine then do so, perhaps at a more gentle rate and try to build slower next time or change what aspects of the exercise you increase

- To be effective your exercise needs to be steady and sustained. If you can only do a few minutes on the first day, that is absolutely great, it's all progress in the right direction.

- When you start your programme, build up to a 10-minute bout at a steady and sustained pace. Then go to 20 minutes, then 30, and ultimately aim for 45–60 minutes. You will soon find it easy to sustain this level of exercise.

- Ideally you do need a bit of 'huff and puff', but you should still be able to hold a conversation while you exercise, otherwise you may well be overdoing things. Working from the continuum as shown below, aim for a level of about 6 or 7.

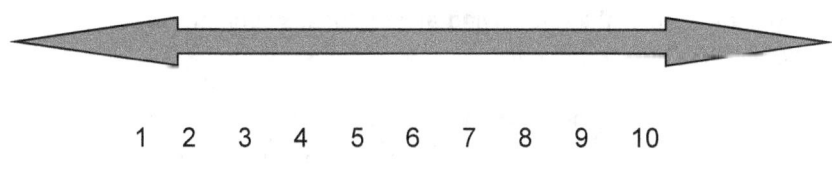

1 2 3 4 5 6 7 8 9 10

RESTING   MILD EXERTION   HIGH EXERTION

Types of activity

Home-based

Your body is a natural weight to exercise against and it doesn't cost you anything. Use what's in your home to exercise — chairs, stairs, walls, floor space. You could also borrow some exercise books from the library, or hire an exercise dvd.

Of course, gardening and housework can burn up a fair few calories as well!

Gym-based

Most gyms provide a wide range of facilities. Many offer a free trial visit so do go along and have a look around and test out the classes or gym equipment to see if this is for you.

- For weightlifting you can use machines, or lift free weights.
- For cardiovascular training you can walk or run on the treadmill; use the cross trainer or stepping machine or use the rowing machine.
- You can do a variety of exercise on a large Swiss ball, which is great for muscle strengthening.
- If you enjoy group fitness then try out some of the many classes on offer such as zumba, step, dance or body pump. Work at your own level and don't feel you have to stay for the whole class.

Pool-based

Consider some of the following at your local swimming pool:

- Aqua jogging allows you to walk/ jog while buoyed by the water, which takes the stress off your joints. It's also great for pregnant women, older people, very overweight people or those with weak joints.
- Pool walking – many pools these days now have a lane for very slow swimmers or walkers.

- Once you're used to walking you may wish to progress to kicking lengths using a flutter board, playing in the pool, or swimming breast stroke, back stroke or freestyle
- Aqua aerobics classes are also a good way to build your water confidence and this is a great form of gentle exercise.

Outdoors

Outdoors is a great place to exercise. Go for a walk in the countryside or along the beach; go cycling or jogging; or have a look at getting involved in activities such as golf. There are many options for exercising either solo or with groups of people if you'd like to combine socialising with some physical activity!

Staying safe

It is important to exercise safely at all times. Wear the correct clothing and footwear; if cycling wear a helmet; always wear a hat and sunscreen in the summer when outdoors, and keep well-hydrated.

Activity and weight management

Ideally we should all aim for at least 30 minutes of exercise every day; but when we are aiming to reduce our weight it is even better if we can more than this. Aim to build up slowly to at least 60 minutes of activity on most, if not all, days of the week and do a mix of aerobic, strength and flexibility exercises. As well as having regular exercise, remember to move more and sit less, being as active as you can in your daily life.

By increasing the amount of energy we are burning off, and reducing the amount of energy we are consuming, we can effectively reduce our body weight and improve our overall health and well-being.

6 FOOD AND BEHAVIOUR

Have you ever thought seriously about the situations that trigger your need to eat? Do you always feel hungry when you eat; or are there other reasons for eating?

It's important to learn to recognise hunger — that growly, empty feeling in your stomach — rather than following other cues. Realise there is a difference between being 'hungry' and just wanting to eat food for reasons other than hunger.

Palatability

Do you often eat simply because the food looks and tastes good? If you weren't hungry and were offered a bowl of raw vegetables, would you decline? What about if you were offered a bowl of chocolates — could you resist? Think about whether your eating is driven by internal signals, such as hunger, or external signals such as the palatability of food. If you can educate yourself to eat only when you're hungry, this can help in the control of your weight.

Emotional eating

Emotional reasons for eating may include feeling depressed, bored, tired or stressed. When feelings other than hunger lead you to overeat; think about what under-pins your overeating and then come up with strategies to deal with the issue without turning to food.

Depressed or anxious

Depression and anxiety can lead to overeating and weight gain. Feeling stressed, miserable or sad now and again is a normal part of life for most people. However if you feel intense and constant unhappiness you may be depressed; and if you feel constant worry or tension, especially in the absence of any particular cause, you may have a generalised anxiety disorder. If you think depression and/or anxiety may be an issue for you it is important to see your GP for a proper medical assessment and for recommendations on treatment. Medication and/or counselling may be recommended, along with dietary therapy and lifestyle interventions.

Research into diet and mental health is ongoing; but recent research has shown that healthy diets consisting of vegetables, fruits, beef, lamb and wholegrains, have been associated with a lower likelihood of depressive and anxiety disorders; whereas a 'Western-pattern' diet, comprising foods such as processed, fatty and sugary foods such as chips, processed meats, meat pies, white breads, hamburgers, sugar, flavoured milk, pizza and beer, have been associated with a higher likelihood of psychological symptoms and disorders.

Whether you are a bit down or clinically depressed; getting on track with the right diet and lifestyle is very likely to help your recovery. Eating a good healthy diet will help you feel better and will help you manage your weight.

Stressed

The pressures today on how we perform and how we look are immense. Being pulled in all directions can cause a considerable amount of stress, and one of the ways we cope is by seeking release in food. Usually we just reach for the nearest convenient food, which is often a chocolate bar, lollies or biscuits. Have you noticed too that often you don't even taste or notice what you're eating? Sometimes it can be quite a shock to realise that you've polished off a packet of biscuits while you were fretting. If you recognise that stress is making you overeat, you can address the underlying problem. Stress often occurs when we have too much to do and feel we are losing control of our lives. If you feel you are losing control, it's time to sit back and take stock. Is there anything you can do to get better organised? Is there anyone else who can help you — family, partner, friends, neighbours? Can you cut down your hours at work, or possibly get a cleaner to take some pressure off at home?

Often we are so busy that we put our own needs last, after everyone else's. It's important to have some **'you'** time, whether this is half an hour each morning with a meditation tape, a couple of trips a week to the gym, or even a facial once a month.

Tired

Tiredness and fatigue are common in this day and age. Many of us are struggling to juggle the demands of modern day life, managing work, family commitments and other obligations. All too often tiredness can lead to overeating as a coping mechanism. Try not to overdo things and recognise your limitations. Think about managing your time effectively and factor in some time for yourself where you just relax or do something enjoyable.

Find other ways to deal with tiredness and fatigue other than overeating and ensure you are having a healthy balanced diet that provides all the nutrients you need for good health. This way your body will be operating at optimal capacity and you will be firing on all cylinders.

Bored or lonely

Have you noticed that the urge to eat is exacerbated if you're bored? Learn to recognise this and do something about it. There's nothing like being busy to take the focus off food, so look for things to occupy you so that you can't eat at the same time. For example, why not try:

- A dance group — ceroc, rock and roll, Latin American.
- Yoga or meditation classes.
- Helping out at school or playgroup.
- A night class.
- Joining a gym.
- Self-defence classes.
- Joining (or forming) a book club.
- Pampering yourself.

- Read a book.
- Have a bubble bath.
- Go to the movies.
- Meet a friend for coffee.
- Take a walk in the countryside.

Keeping a food diary

To understand the cues to eating, why not keep a diary? This a great starting point and enables you to evaluate your current habits objectively, which will then enable you to plan the changes you want to make.

Buy a pocket notebook and write down when you eat, what you eat and how you're feeling at the time, as shown in the following example:

For this to work you need to be honest with yourself: write down everything, it all counts. Stick to your normal habits, so you can figure out where you're at; don't change what you are eating just because you are writing it down. Record things as you go, rather than relying on memory. Be specific about what you have eaten and how you're feeling. Once you have a good record of your own personal reasons for eating, you can begin to address the issues in your life.

Key things to remember are:

- Write down everything including meals, snacks, treats and drinks.
- Write down the quantities so you can monitor changes in food intake, for example in weight, or in cups or in tablespoons/teaspoons.
- Include the method of cooking such as baking or frying
- Include additions to a food such as sugar, grated cheese, salt, oil, soy sauce, other sauces or spreads.
- Include extra remarks such as whether you are eating out or at home, whether you are generally well or ill (with an infection), how you are feeling

and any relevant stressful events that may have influenced your eating patterns.

Here is a Food Diary template that you can use as a starting point. Use this template to record your food intake. Try to do this for at least three days and include one weekend day.

FOOD	TIME	FOOD EATEN	REMARKS

Food addiction

There has been much in the way of research in recent years into food addiction and it is a topic of ongoing research and debate. But how do you know if you are addicted to food?

Try answering the following to help you decide if food addiction is a problem for you. If you have answered yes to **two** or more of the following questions then you may have a food addiction.

- Do you need to consume increasing amounts of foods to satisfy yourself and to achieve a feeling of fullness?
- Do you feel distressed or depressed when you try to reduce your food intake?
- Do you consume larger amounts of food than you intended to on a regular basis?
- Do you experience a lack of success when you try to curtail the amount of food you eat?
- Do you experience a persistent desire for food in excess of your energy requirements?
- Do you spend a great deal of your time eating more than you should?
- Do you maintain your habit of over-eating despite adverse psychological or physical consequences?
- Does over-eating get in the way of your work or spending time with family and friends.

NEEDNT foods

A research paper published in the New Zealand Medical Journal in February 2012[1] listed a selection of foods that

---

[1] Elmslie JD, Sellman JD, Schroder RN et al (2012). The NEEDNT food list: non-essential, energy-dense, nutritionally-deficient foods. NZ Med J 125: 84-92.

the researchers have described as NEEDNT (non-essential, energy-dense nutritionally deficient) foods. The NEEDNT foods list was formulated in response to growing evidence that the emotional and addictive components of overeating need to be addressed for people struggling with overweight and obesity. If you have a problem with food addiction then this list can be a useful tool in replacing the foods that lead you to over-eat with healthier alternatives. Have a look at the list and see if some of the suggestions would be helpful to you

Table 6: The NEEDNT food list

NEEDNT FOOD	REPLACE WITH:
1. Alcoholic drinks	Water/diet soft drinks
2. Biscuits	*
3. Butter, lard, dripping or similar fat (used as a spread or in baking/cooking etc.)	Lite margarine or similar spread or omit
4. Cakes	*
5. Chocolate	*
6. Coconut cream	Lite coconut milk/coconut flavoured lite evaporated milk
7. Condensed milk	*
8. Cordial	Water/Sugar free cordial
9. Corn chips	*
10. Cream (including crème fraiche)	Natural yoghurt (or flavoured yoghurt depending on use)
11. Crisps (including vegetable crisps)	*
12. Desserts/puddings	*
13. Doughnuts	*
14. Drinking Chocolate,	Cocoa plus artificial

Milo etc.	sweetener
15. Energy drinks	Water
16. Flavoured milk/milkshakes	Trim, Calcitrim or Lite Blue Milk
17. Fruit tinned in syrup (even lite syrup!)	Fruit tinned in juice/artificially sweetened
18. Fried food	Boiled, grilled or baked food
19. Frozen yoghurt	Ordinary yoghurt
20. Fruit juice (except tomato juice and unsweetened blackcurrant juice)	Fresh fruit (apple, orange, pear etc. + a drink!)
21. Glucose	Artificial sweetener
22. High fat crackers (≥ 10g fat per 100g)	Lower fat crackers (≤ 10g fat per 110g)
23. Honey	*
24. Hot chips	*
25. Ice cream	*
26. Jam	*
27. Marmalade	*
28. Mayonnaise	Lite dressings/lite mayonnaise
29. Muesli bars	*

30. Muffins   *

31. Nuts roasted in fat or oil   Dry roasted or raw nuts (≤ 1 handful per day)

32. Pastries   *

33. Pies   *

34. Popcorn with butter or oil   Air popped popcorn

35. Quiches   Crust-less quiches

36. Reduced cream   Natural yoghurt

37. Regular luncheon sausage   Low fat luncheon sausage

38. Regular powdered drinks (e.g. Raro)   Water/Diet/Sugar free powdered drinks

39. Regular salami   Low fat salami

40. Regular sausages   Low fat sausages

41. Regular soft drinks   Water/Diet soft drinks

42. Rollups   Fresh fruit

43. Sour cream   Natural yoghurt

44. Sugar (added to anything including drinks, baking, cooking etc.)   Artificial sweetener

45. Sweets/lollies   *

46. Syrups such as golden syrup, treacle, maple syrup   Artificial sweetener

47. Toasted muesli and any other breakfast cereal with ≥ 15g sugar per 100g cereal	Breakfast cereal with <15g sugar per 100g cereal, > 6g fibre per 100g cereal and <5g fat per 100g cereal (or <10 g fat per 100g cereal if cereal contains nuts and seeds)
48. Whole Milk	Trim, Calcitrim or Lite Blue Milk
49. Yoghurt type products with ≥ 10g sugar per 100g yoghurt	Yoghurt (not more than one a day)

Here are some other suggestions for replacing some of the common foods that people can be addicted to:

- Chocolate cravings: have a low-calorie hot chocolate drink made with trim milk instead, or the occasional small portion of low-fat chocolate ice cream.
- If you feel you just really need to eat chocolate – pop along to your local dairy once a week and just buy a single mini-chocolate bar such as a Freddo frog.
- Sweet cravings: have sugar-free chewing gum instead.
- Potato chip cravings: have popcorn instead – but make sure it is the home made variety which is easy to make in the microwave and don't add any extra fat, salt or sugar.
- Cheese cravings: try the low-fat varieties instead. Buy much smaller quantities, grate and sprinkle it over food as flavouring rather than serving large amounts.

Mindfulness and food

Being mindful around food is another strategy than can help with reducing your food intake. Research suggests that people who are mindful around food can more successfully manage their weight. Being mindful in relation to food involves the following:

- **Eat slowly.** Chew more slowly, take breaks between bites of food, be aware of whether you are getting full and have had enough food. Take a break part way through a meal or snack, take some deep breaths an assess how you feel.

- **Utilise your senses.** Really **observe** the **taste**, **smell** and **texture** of the food you are eating.

- **Focus on the food.** Try not to let your mind get distracted.

- **Eat away from distractions.** Don't eat while watching TV, working, sitting at the computer, or while driving or travelling in the car.

- **Become aware of hunger and fullness cues.** Use these cues to make decisions about when to eat and how much to eat.

- **Acknowledge responses to food in a non-judgemental way**. Observe how you feel about different food choices – what you like, what you dislike and what you're neutral about.

- **Choose to eat foods that are both pleasing and nourishing.** In other words, choose foods that have a high nutritional value and that you like to eat because of the taste, smell, texture or colour.

- **Reflect on your feelings around eating.** You might find yourself eating **unmindfully** and feeling happy, sad, bored or guilty around eating; reflect on the effects of eating in this way. If you have been eating inappropriate or unhealthy foods In excessive amounts you might experience the physical effects of bloating, discomfort, heartburn or indigestion. Think about how you might make different choices in the future.

- **Remember the five Ds,** if you feel the urge to over-eat the wrong kinds of food:

  - **DELAY** reaching for the food
  - Take a **DEEP** breath
  - Have a **DRINK** of water
  - **DISTRACT** yourself with another activity
  - If you're genuinely hungry, **DIVERT** your attention by having a healthy snack such as some fruit.

Planning for change

Where are you currently?

Are you ready to make changes and eager to get started or does it all seem too hard? If you are still struggling with the idea of getting started why not write down a list of reasons why you want to make changes. For example:

- To improve your health and well-being.
- To prevent or manage chronic diseases such as diabetes or cardiovascular disease.
- To feel better about yourself and improve your confidence levels.
- To fit into your old clothes.
- To have more energy to enjoy life, manage workloads and socialise with friends and family.
- To be a great role model for your children.

We are all at different stages of our lives and have different priorities so sit down and have a think about what will really motivate you to get started and to stick with it.

Too busy to bother?

One of the most common barriers to making changes is being busy. Many of us lead very busy lives these days juggling lots of responsibilities and it can be hard to make time to shop for, prepare and eat healthy foods. This means we often end up eating on the run and grabbling whatever is to hand at the time – and this might not be the best choice for our health and for managing our weight.

The key really is to get organised. If you have a busy job prepare a healthy packed lunch the night before. Pack up some healthy snacks too to take along to work. If you are a busy Mum with young children – do sit down and eat with the kids and role model good food habits for them to follow. All to often as Mums we are so busy running around after the rest of the family and making sure their needs are met that we don't properly look after ourselves and habits such as grazing, snacking and ultimately over-eating can set in without us even realising it.

So, just remember these key points and you will be on the right track:

- Make the healthy option the easy option; always make sure you have healthy food on hand at home and at work.
- Shop wisely, ensure a healthy shopping list and stick to it.
- Take packed meals and snacks to work if necessary.
- Prepare healthy snacks for home and keep them in the fridge and store cupboard.

Goal setting

It is important to set small achievable goals so you don't set yourself up for failure. Think about setting **SMART** goals; which are specific, measureable, achievable, relisting and time focussed. Here are some examples of the types of things that you might like to consider when setting SMART goals.

SPECIFIC:

For example 'I will eat five portions of fruits and vegetables each day'.

MEASURABLE:

The goals will be ones that can be measured; for example 'I will go for a 30 minute walk each day', or 'I will eat a piece of fruit with lunch each day'.

ACHIEVABLE:

You are much more likely to be able to stick to goals that are achievable. If you goal is to eat less fat then look at ways of progressing towards this goal, for example changing from whole milk to a lower fat milk (light blue, or green top), only buying lean meat, having low fat oven chips instead of fried chips.

REALISTIC:

Don't set yourself up for disappointment. If you aim to lose 5kg in a week you will fail. Set small achievable goals such as 'I will aim to lose 5-10% of my body weight in total'; 'I will aim to lose 0.5kg a week'.

TIME FOCUSED:

Set a time period by which you will achieve your goals; for example you may have short term goals such as eating an extra piece of fruit a day which you will achieve in a week. You may also have longer term goals, for example to lose 12kg in 6 months.

MY TOP THREE SMART GOALS:

Now, set yourself three SMART goals by filling in the boxes.

NUMBER	GOAL
1	
2	
3	

Overcoming setbacks

We are human as we can al have set backs no matter how determined we are to follow a healthy diet. It may be that you become ill; or go on holiday; or are invited to a dinner party and don't want to offend your host.

Don't be too hard on yourself, and when you do have a set back just aim to get back on track as soon as possible.

Diets always begin tomorrow, so the saying goes, but there's no time like the present to start making changes that will be of such great benefit in the longer term. The trick to implementing a new healthy eating plan is working out which changes in diet and activity will work for you. The starting point might be to just carry on as you are for a week while recording your feelings. It might be, however, that you are keen to get straight into a whole new lifestyle. The important thing is to begin the changes now, and to ensure that they are easy, achievable, and enjoyable, and therefore sustainable.

Self monitoring

Self monitoring can be a helpful way of keeping on track.

Record your food intake (see the section on keeping a food diary); record your activity levels on a daily basis to make sure you aren't slipping; and keep a note of your body measurements such as weight and waist measurement. By keeping a record you can look back and assess what was working when you were successfully reducing your weight and what was happening when you were maintaining (or even gaining) weight. This will help you to highlight strategies for success.

Rewarding achievements

Did you resist the jam doughnut at the cake shop? Did you choose a herbal tea instead of an iced chocolate with cream at the café? Have you managed to substitute unhealthy foods such as chippies and chocolates for healthier snacks such as fruit and vegetables?

Take a moment to congratulate yourself and focus on your achievements? Having planned rewards can be motivating and inspiring too – for example buying some new clothes, going for a massage or treating yourself to a new book or CD.

It is important to recognise the great achievement of making and sustaining changes in your life; this will help you to stay focussed on your goals.

Planning ahead for risky situations

We often find ourselves in situations that are challenging. For example:

- Going to a friend's house for dinner and not wanting to make a fuss.
- Going away on a business trip and only having hotel/restaurant food available.
- Going on holiday with family or friends
- Attending work social functions or meetings
- Attending conferences where there are set meals and snacks

Have a think about how you will deal with different situations to make sure you do not over-eat. For example you might like to have a healthy snack before attending a social function or morning tea at work – if you aren't hungry you will be less likely to snack on the pies, pastries, sausage rolls or muffins that are so often served on these types of occasions.

If you are going to a friends house you may tell them you are following a special diet – or if you feel uncomfortable with that you could just say when you get there that you aren't very hungry and could you just have a small portion of food.

Hotels and restaurants will often cater for special diets – so do ask if they can swap the fries for a salad, or provide you with a starter sized portion, or adapt what is on the menu so it better suits you needs.

Conferences are tricky – especially if they go on all day, as there is often a full programme and not enough opportunity to leave the venue. As such, you really have to just eat what's there. However; you could always just have a drink and steer clear of unhealthy snacks during the morning and afternoon tea breaks – and lunches are often buffet style lunches so you can serve yourself smaller amounts of food. Just remember too, if you do over-eat a bit for one day, you can always get right back on track as soon as the conference is over.

Holidays just often involve planning ahead. Are you staying in a motel and able to shop for and prepare your own food? If so that means you will have more control over what you are eating. If the food is supplied by a hotel have a chat with the catering staff about serving foods that will best meet your needs. And if staying with family or friends, do let them know that you are following a healthy eating plan – you may even be able to get them on board with it too!

Social support

Having good support networks can be helpful when you are managing your weight. Family/whānau, friends, and colleagues can all help to maintain your motivation and provide positive reinforcement. Involve your partners if possible – they may even want to get on board with you as you start your healthy eating regimen. Whether or not the rest of the family need to lose weight, you will all benefit from having a healthy balanced diet. If the rest of the family are a healthy eight then you will just be tweaking back your portions a little at the dinner table to reduce your energy intake and promote weight loss.

7 PUTTING IT ALL TOGETHER

So remember, it's all about food, activity and behaviour. Here is a summary of some of the key points to think about when you are reducing your weight.

Food

- Have appropriate portion sizes – with smaller amounts when following a healthy weight-reducing diet.
- Have an increased daily intake of fruits and vegetables.
- Go for wholegrains and other low GI/high fibre foods.
- Reduce total fat intake.
- When you do eat fat – choose the healthier monounsaturated and polyunsaturated fatty acids.
- Avoid where possible any foods that contain saturated and *trans* fatty acids.
- Choose the lower-fat dairy products.
- Choose lean cuts of meat.
- Remove skin from poultry and trim all visible fat from meat.
- Include nuts in the diet (in moderation) as a healthy snack.
- Have a regular intake of fish.
- Steer clear, as much as possible, from the high-fat unhealthy take-away foods, fast foods and fried foods.
- Reduce as much as possible intake of energy-dense foods such as potato chips, pies and pastries, biscuits, ice-cream, lollies, buttered popcorn, cakes and chocolates.
- Limit intake of sugary drinks such as fizzy drinks, fruit juices, energy drinks and flavoured cordial drinks.
- Learn to read food labels so you can make better food choices.
- Don't deny yourself your favourite foods – nothing is banned from your diet – it is all about how much you eat and how often. By having a little treat now and again you will reduce the risk of bingeing on the wrong foods.

- Do keep yourself away from foods that tempt you. Try not to have them in the house. At parties steer clear of the buffet table and socialise away from the food.

Activity

- Start slowly with any new exercise regimen.
- Build up from 5-10 minutes of activity per day if you have not been active to date.
- If it's easier, break down activity into smaller bouts throughout the day.
- The ideal amount of activity for successful weight loss **is 60 minutes per day.**
- Reduce sedentary leisure time (e.g. watching TV, sitting at the computer, playing video games).
- Be active in as many ways as possible – in your work life, your leisure time and your travelling (e.g. walk or ride a bike instead of driving or taking a bus).
- Include physical activity in your daily life where ever possible – for example take the stairs instead of the lift, where possible, get up from your desk and walk over to talk to someone instead of emailing or calling on the phone.
- Consider exercising with a friend or getting involved in group based activities.
- Include muscle strengthening activities on **at least two days a week.**
- Ensure you exercise regularly but don't over-do it.

Behaviour

- Recruit your friends, family, and spouse into supporting you in your weight loss programme.
- Write down what you eat and drink during the day and when and record thoughts and feelings so you can identify strategies to change your behaviour around food.
- Be 'mindful' around food and eat slowly. Take time away from other activities to enjoy your meals and snacks.

- A healthy weight loss diet is the same as a healthy weight maintenance, diet but with reduced portions – so your meal patterns will be suitable for the whole family.
- Identify areas you would like to approach first (for example – food or activity).
- Set small achievable goals.
- Use problem solving technique and incremental goal setting strategies, for example walking for five minutes a day and increasing by five minutes at the end of each week.
- Identify activities you find enjoyable – make a list of 10 fun activities that you like to do (that don't revolve around food) – reading a book, watching a movie, having a long soak in the bath, walking at the beach, meditating, listening to music. When you are bored, stressed or fed-up choose an activity other than food to keep you occupied. Food should be fuel, not entertainment or emotional fulfilment.
- Treat un-met goals as challenges and the opportunity to understand your own barriers to success and how to over come these.
- If you are struggling to keep to a weight loss plan – don't be too hard on yourself. Give yourself a day off each week and relax!

Maintaining weight loss

When you reach your goals, aim for **Weight-Loss Maintenance** as there is nothing more disheartening than re-gaining weight that you have worked so hard to lose.

To successfully ensure **Weight-Loss Maintenance**, you'll still need to adopt the strategies discussed in this book. You should still be following a healthy eating plan – but you will be able to nudge up the portion sizes a little so you are maintaining and not losing weight. Keep an eye on your weight and if it starts to creep up – even by as little as 2kg, then get straight back on your weight reducing diet. Keep exercising too – physical activity is an important part of weight maintenance.

In summary

- Ensure you have a weight maintenance programme in place.
- Monitor your weight weekly.
- If a weight re-gain of 1.5-2kg occurs, recommence your weight-reducing plan immediately.
- Maintain a healthy diet and at least 30-45mins of activity every day.

The End

ABOUT THE AUTHOR

The Kiwi Nutrition weight management guide has been carefully put together by nutritionist Amanda Johnson.

Amanda has a long standing interest and many years experience helping people change the way they eat to improve their health. She was previously the Executive Director of the New Zealand Dietetic Association and has also been PR Officer and media spokesperson for the British Dietetic Association. In addition, she has recently worked for New Zealand's Science Media Centre, focussing on health and nutrition issues.

As a specialist in weight management, Amanda has helped many people internationally and, more recently, across the Wellington region, achieve substantial nutrition weight-loss goals in her private clinical practice.

She is the author of The Power of Positive Eating, a New Zealand guide to weight loss, and editor of the British Nutrition Foundation Task Force Report on Obesity, a scientific report written by some of the world's leading experts in obesity. She is also co-author of Nutrition – a Handbook for Community Nurses. In addition, she has recently written scientific reports on the role of seafood in a healthy New Zealand diet and on the role of red meat in a healthy New Zealand diet. She is also a frequent media commentator on food-related issues.

Copyright

No part of this information guide may be reproduced, forwarded, photocopied or transmitted in any form, or by any means, unless with written permission from the author.

© Amanda Johnson 2015.